Blessings

FAITH IN BROKEN PLACES

Understanding God's Plan in the Midst of Pain

by Bestselling Author
Kim Brooks

Faith in Broken Places
Understanding God's Plan in the Midst of Pain

http://www.KimOnTheWeb.com

All Scripture quotations, unless otherwise indicated, are from the
Holy Bible, King James Version.

All definitions, unless otherwise indicated, are from the Strong's
Concordance.

ISBN: 0976039052
ISBN 13: 9780976039051

ACKNOWLEDGEMENTS

I would like to thank God and the many family members (biological and spiritual), friends and loved ones who took the time out to pray for me, visit me in the hospital, call or text, bring food or just sit with me to enjoy laughter and fellowship during a very difficult time in my life. I will forever remember you and your selfless acts of love. God is truly faithful, and I pray my testimony blesses and encourages you in the midst of whatever you may be going through right now. God is the mender of all brokenness, and as long as you continue to keep your mind stayed on Him, you will soon step into your place of victory on the other side (so shout right now!) Hallelujah!

DEDICATION

This book is dedicated to the loving memory of my beautiful mom, Lutricia Brooks, who, while this book was being published, made her transition to be with the Lord. To be absent from the body means to be present with Him, and I have peace knowing right now she is singing and dancing in heaven. Thank you, Jesus!

CHAPTER 1
THE ACCIDENT

Thursday, April 9

I can remember it like it was yesterday, though it happened almost a month ago on March 14 – twenty-six days, or 627½ hours ago to be exact. It was the day I was involved in a very bad car accident; it was the day that changed my life forever.

"Your femur bone was broken in three places," the doctor told me.

"What?" I thought to myself. *"You have got to be kidding me."* Unfortunately the X-rays confirmed it.

I should've known it was serious after experiencing excruciating pain while nurses shifted my body from the hospital bed to the X-ray table.

"JESUS!" I screamed at the top of my lungs.

It probably scared the living bejeebies out of everyone in the room.

I could tell by their faces they couldn't understand why I screamed so much, until finally one doctor had enough common sense to check the IV in my arm containing the morphine. It was swollen, which meant the IV wasn't inserted in my vein properly which meant all pain – I could feel.

So I wasn't just some nut screaming in the X-ray room; my screams were warranted.

Thanks to my mother, whom I love dearly, my veins are extremely small. By the time I left the hospital two weeks later my arms had so many pokes in them from their trying to find good veins that one would think I was a victim of domestic violence.

Not to mention the bruises on my right arm and left hand that weren't tended to. It wasn't major, nothing a little Neosporin couldn't handle – I guess in all the hustle and bustle the doctors and nurses instead had to focus what was really important: my leg.

So back to the night of the accident; after the X-rays and the horrible dreaded news, I was told not to drink any liquids in preparation for surgery first thing in the morning. Then, as I finally settled in a room, another doctor said my surgery wouldn't be until two days later on Monday.

"What?"

Thankfully, once I complained about how I was told surgery was in the morning and not the following day, which was why I hadn't had so much as a sip of water, I received an update that my surgery will indeed be first thing in the morning at 7 a.m. Thank you, Lord.

Prayer works.

Surgery went well; they put a rod in my leg and told me over time, with the assistance of physical therapy, it will heal.

I was blessed beyond measure by the overflow of love and support as around the clock the day following the surgery and beyond, family, friends and loved ones flooded my room with flowers, cards, prayers, and encouragement.

I had no idea I was so loved; and I must admit it was a great feeling.

Here I am thinking all I would see following the surgery were my mother and sister Kelley, yet I've seen so many more, and even now I still get calls and visits from loved ones expressing their care and concern.

It definitely feels good to be cared about; that's the one good thing I can say about this whole episode. People are God's way of expressing His love for us on the earth; which led me to believe that maybe, in the midst of all this pain, maybe God does care.

I'll admit, during this whole thing, I've had my good days and my bad days.

Anyone who would talk to me would swear that I was in great spirits and coming along just fine. What they failed to realize is that the reason I was in great spirits was because I was genuinely happy to be talking to *them*. They were the ones who put me in great spirits in the first place – simply by calling, simply by stopping by, simply by caring.

I'm an extrovert by nature, and while many believe to be an extrovert means to be an outgoing social butterfly, it actually is a description of where one draws one's energy from. Extroverts draw their energy from people, where introverts draw theirs from within. I'm energized and bubbly around people because being around them makes me happy. I love people, and am genuinely interested in what they have to say. The major challenge with extroverts, though, is when the lights are off and everyone's gone, the extrovert is left to deal with himself or herself – and unless you have a friend named Jesus, being alone can be a very lonely place.

Case in point – the first week after leaving the hospital, at night at my place I was very uneasy. It was almost as if I was getting used to living alone all over again, like I hadn't lived on my own for the last ten years.

I guess being cooped up in a hospital for two weeks, one week in the trauma unit and the other week for rehab and three hours a day worth of physical therapy, caused me to be excited upon leaving, yet anxious about going from seemingly one den hole to another.

That's the worst part about this whole thing; being stuck in the apartment day after day after day.

Today was eventful, though, I actually had two doctor's appointments – one a follow-up appointment with my surgeon and the other an appointment to confirm home safety and medical equipment needs. I was out almost all day today, and though it was dreary and raining (even now there's a thunderstorm watch) I still felt like a kid out to a candy store.

It was not until after having a serious car accident did I realize how something as simple as fresh air can be a tremendous gift.

And how something as simple as walking is not a right, but a privilege.

I look forward to the day I can walk again, and though therapists seem to have full faith that I will be able to walk again real soon, with each passing day I wonder if it will be so as I tire of traveling with a walker or wheelchair to and fro.

"It'll get better," I must tell myself. I must believe it.

CHAPTER 2

FAITH WHEN IT'S HARD TO BELIEVE

Saturday, April 11

Faith is an amazing concept.

Scripture tells us in *Hebrews 11:1*:

Now faith is the substance of things hoped for, the evidence of things not seen.

The word, *faith*, in the Bible is translated from the Greek word, *pistis*, which by definition means: conviction of the truth of anything, belief with the predominate idea of trust (or confidence), fidelity or faithfulness, and the character of one who can be relied on.

Admittedly, it's hard to have faith in dark places.

It's hard to have faith in places where you can't see.

It's hard to have faith when folk tell you it could take anywhere from six weeks to up to two years for a fractured femur bone, the longest and strongest bone in one's leg, to heal.

It's hard to have faith when you're told either your bone will grow additional bone around itself and heal it, or it won't and you could be in excruciating pain for the rest of your life.

It's hard to have faith when you can't immediately see the outcome, and when you don't always understand.

It's hard, but it's necessary.

It's necessary in order to not only survive, but thrive.

. . . the just shall live by faith . . . Hebrews 10:38

While I've never considered myself as one who plays the victim, I will admit tonight I had a bit of a pity party earlier while asking God, *"Why?"*

No, it wasn't the typical, *"Why me, Lord?"* I figured a car accident could happen to anyone, and that I was no exception. But one thing I did cry out and ask God, with tears streaming down my face, was, *"Why didn't You protect me, Lord?"*

Here I am, living for God, loving and worshiping Him and wanting to do nothing more than to serve Him and be a blessing to His people, yet an all-knowing, all-seeing and all-powerful God allowed this tragic accident to happen.

Not only did He allow it to happen, I was an eyewitness to the whole thing.

As I headed south on John R Road in Hazel Park, MI, following praise team rehearsal and a church meeting, and headed home while minding my own business, I literally saw the other driver pull out of a side street without stopping at the stop sign and turn left right into me. It was as if I were invisible to him.

While I swerved in an attempt to get away, it was too late. We collided, and my car catapulted to the other side of the road, front windows smashed, air bag deployed, car totaled.

All I could remember was screaming, "My leg! My leg!" As I reached in my purse on the passenger seat and dialed 911, a good Samaritan, a young blond girl in a red pea coat, grabbed my phone out of my hand, talked to the police and then called my mom to tell her I had been involved in an accident.

I believe the other driver was injured as well, but while he walked out of his car, I had to be gurneyed out.

Conscious the whole time, as I headed to Beaumont Hospital in Royal Oak, MI, the nice, handsome officer who rode with me comforted me with his words during the trip. He asked me if he could do anything, and without hesitation I simply asked him to hold my hand, which he lovingly obliged.

With all this I did wonder, *"Where were my angels, Lord?"*

We sing about Jesus being a fence of protection all around us every day, but where was my fence on Saturday, March 14, 2015?

It's hard to have faith when you don't always understand.

However in order to keep my sanity and peace of mind, I must believe and be fully persuaded that God loves me in the midst of all of this.

I must have confidence in the God who created the earth, the stars and the moon and in the God who created me.

He said I am wonderfully and fearfully made *(Psalm 139:14)* so I must believe that the God who made me can also repair me if I'm broken.

I must believe that not only is He the mender of the brokenhearted, but that He is also the mender of all brokenness.

He created our hearts, He created our minds, He created our bodies and He created our bones, so if the goal is for God to create more bone to grow around the rod in order to reconnect and heal it, then so be it – I must believe it.

Even when it's hard to believe, I must stand up to myself and tell myself I must believe.

Either I believe, or I die.

. . . the just shall live by faith . . .

CHAPTER 3
I'VE COME TOO FAR

Sunday, April 12

In the midst of my temper tantrum as I asked God why He didn't protect me, the following is His response:

I protect you.
I protect you every day.
I'm protecting you now . . .
just continue to have faith
and trust in Me.

Faith.

Conviction.

Belief with the prominent idea of trust or confidence.

Fidelity or faithfulness.

The character of one who can be relied upon.

I must have faith in God's faithfulness.

God has never failed me up until this point, and He won't fail me now.

I've come too far for Him to leave me, and He already said in His Word that He will never leave me nor forsake me *(Hebrews 13:5)*.

He has healed me before, and He can be relied upon to heal me again.

I must believe it.

I must receive it.

Not only in my mind, but in my heart and in my soul.

I must have faith in His promises to me.

I must have faith in them every single day.

CHAPTER 4
SOUL FOOD

Wednesday, April 15

S o today was a positive day.

I Googled foods that heal broken bones in order to, along with prayer, promote a speedy recovery – at least as speedy as possible. I discovered foods high in calcium such as fat free or skim milk, yogurt and cheese help along with leafy green vegetables like kale, turnip and collard greens, plus Vitamin C foods like oranges, kiwi, tomatoes and papaya. In addition to Vitamin C (I currently take three Vitamin C pills a day), Vitamin K and Vitamin B6 help as well.

But the thing that gives me the brightest glimmer of hope is when I read the following in a report I found online entitled *How To Speed Fracture Healing* by Dr. Susan E. Brown, PhD, that stated, "Nature…moves swiftly to initiate healing. Guided by a complex intelligence that we do not yet fully understand, bone repairs itself – and over a few months is made whole again. The fracture self-repair process is spontaneous, natural, and seeks no direction from us." While the author uses terms such as "nature" and "complex intelligence" I know and believe in a True and Living God who is the author of the healing process.

As I attended a follow-up appointment yesterday my doctor described how eventually bone will grow around the rod inside my leg, for the purpose of reattaching itself to the broken bone in order to heal it fully. He explained how that is the natural process of healing, or it may choose not to do so. So I'm believing God, of course, for this natural process to take place.

God has told me, on several occasions, that I'm His child, His beloved daughter and precious jewel and even Scripture describes how no good thing will He withhold from them that love Him and how He, as a good Father, gives good gifts to those who ask Him. *(Psalm 84:11* and *Matthew 7:11)*

So I'm asking, God, that you, Jehovah Rapha, the Lord who Heals, will heal my body, heal my broken bones naturally the way that You and only You know how. I pray for a speedy, supernatural recovery and that all will be not only healed but also restored and made whole in the Name of Jesus. I thank You that the God I serve is a loving God, a giving God, a gracious God and a healing God. There is no problem too hard for You and nothing too big for you for with God all things are possible. So, Lord, I put my faith in who You are, knowing that what God has for me, is for me, including my healing today. It is done; it is so; in Jesus' Name. Amen.

Amen.

CHAPTER 5

STANDING UP ON THE
INSIDE

Saturday, April 18

Today was rough. Really rough.
I woke up feeling terrible.

The sunshine outside my window on this Saturday morning didn't help either as I longed for the day that I, too, could once again go outside "and play." On a day typically reserved for dates, errands or spending time having fun with family and friends, here I am stuck inside with no where to go.

I eventually crawled out of bed and somehow made my way over to a folder which held none other than a paper that listed my goals for the remainder of this year. Needless to say this goal sheet was created before my accident. Thoughts of anger flooded my mind as I concluded that as a result of the accident, I won't be able to reach many of the goals on the sheet. Then I thought about my current immobility. I'm used to being on the go – whether it's meetings, speaking engagements or whatever, I'm used to going out whenever I wanted. Now I can't even go to the corner store without someone helping me down the stairs with my walker and wheeling me along.

My caregiver, Ursula, entered my apartment exactly at 9 a.m. right on time as usual. Upon entrance she's usually greeted with a chipper, *"Good morning, Ursula,"* from me, then we chat about current events, Facebook drama, men or our families, but this time, when I greeted her with a dismal *"Hello"* she knew something wasn't quite right this particular morning.

"What's wrong?" she asked.

"Oh nothing," I responded, while staring out the window.

I couldn't quite understand how I was feeling this way – like my whole world had collapsed right in front of me. At least the world as I had once known it had seemingly fallen apart. Lord knows I didn't think I would break my leg before I married and had at least one child. Bearing the burden seemingly alone, though I had several family and friends who continuously reminded me of their love and concern every day by phone, visits or text, was beginning to take its toll on me emotionally.

"I will never leave you nor forsake you," God reminds us in *Hebrews 13:5*. The word, *never*, in the original Greek means certainly not or by no means and the word, *leave*, in the Greek means to give up, not to uphold and to sink. Also, the word, *forsake*, in the Greek means totally abandon, leave helpless or leave surviving.

So in essence God is saying He will certainly not and by no means give up on me or cause me to sink nor will he totally abandon me, leave me helpless or simply surviving.

Lord knows we need Him in order to not just survive, but thrive.

We need Him to be with us in dark places, during dark moments of confusion where we may feel totally abandoned and forsaken, when the truth is, we're not.

When I was involved in that car accident, after I discovered my leg was broken, to be honest I felt forsaken by God.

For a brief moment I thought, here I am, Lord, serving and living for You, one minute I'm at praise team rehearsal getting ready to worship and praise you the next day on Sunday morning, except this time before I could even make it home I'm in the hospital having surgery Sunday morning.

The same leg I would use to praise and worship You exuberantly, to head to the altar with my offering and kneel before You, is the same leg that's now broken and immobile.

Though I can't move at full weight bearing on the outside, I can still praise You on the inside.

Instead of focusing on what I don't have, I have to focus on what I have, which is the focus of *Hebrews 13:5*, the first part which many often fail to recite:

> *Let your conversation be without covetousness; and be content with such things as ye have: for he hath said, I will never leave thee, nor forsake thee.*

Before letting me know He will never leave or forsake me, God wants me to be content or satisfied with what I have.

So though, right now, I may not have the ability to jump up and down in order to praise You, I can still shout with a voice of triumph in order to still get my praise on. Though I may not be able to get my dance on like I may want to in order to praise You, I can still shake a shoulder and give a Holy Ghost bank head bounce in order to give Your name some Glory. Though I may often sit down on the outside, I can stand up on the inside while knowing with You, I am never alone, because You will never abandon me nor leave me helpless. Now that's something to shout about.

I will lift up mine eyes unto the hills, from whence cometh my help. My help cometh from the LORD, which made heaven and earth. Psalm 121:1-2

CHAPTER 6
REST

Thursday, April 23

Couldn't sleep last night. Had a lot on my mind.
I can count on one hand the number of times I
slept all the way through. The next morning, I would
feel like heaven on earth. Most nights I wake up at least
once at around 3 a.m. in order to use the restroom, and
then head off to dreamland. But last night was different. I even tried putting on my infamous meditation music found on YouTube, as they have several for sleeping
aids, but not even that worked. At least this afternoon,
though, I was able to catch up on missed sleep and slept
for hours. I found a meditation video that worked this
time, and after listening to Donnie McClurkin's *"I Trust
You, Lord,"* I turned on the relaxing video and slept for at
least three hours. Lord, it felt good to catch up on much
needed rest.

Today reminded me of God's Word which states,

I will both lay me down in peace, and sleep: for thou, Lord, only makest me dwell in safety. Psalm 4:8

Another word for safety is security.

When we feel safe and secure in God, and when we truly believe everything will be all right is when we are able to lay ourselves down in peace and tranquility and truly sleep.

It wasn't until my accident did I find the true blessing in a full night's rest.

Another favorite Scripture of mine concerning sleep is:

When thou liest down, thou shalt not be afraid: yea, thou shalt lie down, and thy sleep shall be sweet. Proverbs 3:24

Fear is something else that robs us of the blessing of sleep.

When we worry and are fearful of tomorrow and of our future, we rob ourselves of not only sleep, but sweet sleep. God blesses us with sweet sleep as we remain firm and secure trusting in Him.

So no matter what may come our way and no matter the circumstance, though the enemy may come in like a flood we have to trust and believe the Spirit of the Lord will raise up a standard against him (*Isaiah 59:19*). We have to trust and believe in Jehovah Nissi the Lord our Righteousness who will fight our battles (*Exodus 17:15*). We have to be still, on the inside, knowing that He is God and with the

Lord on our side what can man do unto us? *(Psalm 46:10; Romans 8:31)*. We have to know that the battle we may be facing, is not ours to fight but that it's already won because He, the great I AM, holds the outcome *(2 Chronicles 20:15)*.

We have to have faith and trust in this fact because otherwise we could go crazy trusting in our own ability and in our own strength.

God said His strength is made perfect in our weakness, but we have to first acknowledge where we are weak and allow Him to bring strength to our weak places *(2 Corinthians 12:9)*.

Thou wilt keep him in perfect peace, whose mind is stayed on thee: because he trusteth in thee. Isaiah 26:3

CHAPTER 7
CELEBRATING SMALL VICTORIES

Monday, May 4

I know it's been a while since I last checked in. I wanted to share a testimony of sorts. Last night . . . I slept on my side – the side of the recovering leg.

I can remember when I stayed in the hospital the full two weeks and beyond at home all I could do was lie on my back to sleep.

I can also remember when I couldn't even adjust myself in the hospital and the nurses had to shift my body over by way of the blanket underneath me in an attempt to get comfortable. So I went from needing assistance to sleep, to only sleeping on my back, to now being able to comfortably sleep on either side with absolutely no pain.

Oh, and I have another testimony – I'm totally off pain pills!

One thing I said even in the hospital is that I didn't want to be one of those persons who would become addicted to pain pills and have to take them every three and four hours. When I first got in the hospital it seemed like they came around like clockwork with pain pills; it got to the point where I nicknamed one of the head nurses my drug dealer. Then I realized that they do say they should be taken "as needed" so instead of agreeing to take two of them every four hours, I took two in the morning with breakfast, and two at night with dinner. I did that for a few weeks and even after I came home but then I went to one in the morning, and one at night, then just one a day, and now I don't take any at all and today I have absolutely zero pain! To God be the Glory! Now, I don't recommend this to you at home because, as it pertains to medication and what you may be going through, you definitely want to consult with your physician first; I just mainly wanted to share what the Lord did for me.

CHAPTER 8
GRATITUDE

Wednesday, May 6

O ne thing I noticed with this whole ordeal is I'm starting to appreciate little things more. I can recall one morning I just woke up and looked outside my window and said, *"Thank you, Lord, for sunshine."*

I mean, it's a blessing to even see another day. I posted a picture of some little boys from Africa smiling from ear to ear with the caption "Smile! You woke up today." As I found that picture online to post I thought to myself, "Here are these young, precious little boys, living in not so ideal conditions in Africa – yet they're still smiling like they're having the time of their lives." Now that's what I call gratitude.

So one of the things I endeavor to do as a result of this ordeal is to have more gratitude in life about things, about people, about God's blessing whether big or small, about everything.

Tomorrow's not promised, and all the blessings we enjoy right now, including a roof over our heads or even eyes to see and be able to read this book, are all gifts from heaven that should never be taken for granted and always be acknowledged.

God is so faithful that He made sure we had the necessities in life, and even in our bodies so that we can always remember and know that He is God and that He loves us. Oh, how He loves us.

The LORD hath appeared of old unto me, saying, Yea, I have loved thee with an everlasting love: therefore with lovingkindness have I drawn thee. Jeremiah 31:3

Every good gift and every perfect gift is from above, and cometh down from the Father of lights, with whom is no variableness, neither shadow of turning. James 1:17

CHAPTER 9
MORE VICTORIES!

Saturday, May 9

Today marked a milestone for me. I was able to take a shower standing up! I hadn't taken a normal shower since before the accident March 14, and that was because since the accident I could only take showers while sitting down in a medical chair.

I can remember when I couldn't even lift my leg to get inside the shower stall without the assistance of an apparatus called a leg lift . . . now, not only can I get my leg in the shower, I can stand up in the shower. To God be the Glory!

This great news came as a result of a good report I received from my follow-up appointment with my surgeon this past Thursday.

He was able to move my fractured leg around with no pain (by the way, I've been off pain pills for about a week now – woo hoo!) and the X-rays showed signs of healing.

I could actually see where the new bone is starting to form in order to merge with the broken bone. Glo-reh! God is so good, and it's so amazing how He works.

Just like my personal healing is not overnight and is a process, your healing, based on whatever you're going through, may be a process as well.

With each day as I prayed and participated in physical therapy at home with leg lift and bed exercises, and as I ate well and increased my intake of omega 3 enriched foods such as salmon, sardines and more which are good for bones, God was working behind the scenes – healing and simply being who He is.

CHAPTER 10
A SETBACK

Friday, May 15

So today I woke up feeling like crap. Today and yesterday my leg hurt when I woke up. I had stopped taking pain pills altogether for the past week but it looks like I'll have to start taking them again. In the bathroom mirror I looked at myself and honestly felt like a cripple. For some reason all these feelings flooded me today; about how I wish I could do more, especially for my mom who's having heightened health challenges herself, and more for myself, too. Being cooped up at my place makes me feel like a hermit to society and even when I go out it's either to a doctor's appointment or to a physical therapy session.

My first outpatient physical therapy session is today.

I pray it goes well. I'm sure it will; I definitely look forward to getting back on the path to walking regularly again. But what if they find out one of my legs is shorter than the other? I read online that that's happened before after surgery, where one leg is one or two inches longer. What if I won't be able to walk right – ever again? I know, I shouldn't be negative. I must bind these negative thoughts in Jesus' Name . . .

CHAPTER 11
HIS WINGS

Wednesday, May 20

Today during my morning prayer and devotion time I was blessed after reading a commentary on *Psalm 91:4:* The image here is that of an eagle, or maybe a hen – in any case it's a picture of a bird that senses danger and then protectively spreads its wings over its young. An expert on birds once told me that this move is very common. A bird senses the approach of a predator, or the threat of something falling from above, and instinctively spreads out its wings like a canopy. Then the fledglings scuttle underneath for shelter. The move is so instinctive that an adult bird will spread those wings even when no fledglings are around!

And the Psalmist – who has almost surely seen this lovely thing happen – the Psalmist thinks of God.

He will cover you with his pinions, and under his wings you will find refuge. The point is that God is our shelter when the winds begin to howl. The point is that under God's wings we are defended, protected, perfectly safe. The

point is that someone else is in charge. Someone big, strong and experienced. Someone who never goes off duty . . .
 Taken from: Sermon: "The Wings of God"
 by Dr. Cornelius Plantinga, Jr.

He that dwelleth in the secret place of the most High shall abide under the shadow of the Almighty.

I will say of the LORD, He is my refuge and my fortress: my God; in him will I trust.

Surely he shall deliver thee from the snare of the fowler, and from the noisome pestilence.

He shall cover thee with his feathers, and under his wings shalt thou trust: his truth shall be thy shield and buckler.

Thou shalt not be afraid for the terror by night; nor for the arrow that flieth by day;

Nor for the pestilence that walketh in darkness; nor for the destruction that wasteth at noonday.

A thousand shall fall at thy side, and ten thousand at thy right hand; but it shall not come nigh thee.

Only with thine eyes shalt thou behold and see the reward of the wicked.

Because thou hast made the LORD, which is my refuge, even the most High, thy habitation;

There shall no evil befall thee, neither shall any plague come nigh thy dwelling.

For he shall give his angels charge over thee, to keep thee in all thy ways.

They shall bear thee up in their hands, lest thou dash thy foot against a stone.

Thou shalt tread upon the lion and adder: the young lion and the dragon shalt thou trample under feet.

Because he hath set his love upon me, therefore will I deliver him: I will set him on high, because he hath known my name.

He shall call upon me, and I will answer him: I will be with him in trouble; I will deliver him, and honour him.

With long life will I satisfy him, and shew him my salvation.

Psalm 91

CHAPTER 12
A REAL WALK BY FAITH

Sunday, May 24

Wow – this morning I woke up feeling great. I slept all the way through from 11 p.m. to 7 a.m. then went back to sleep and woke up officially at 8:30 am and I kid you not, I feel like the Lord kicked up another notch of healing in my leg last night.

I literally feel like I can walk regularly! Not wanting to go against the doctor's orders, as he currently has me on 50% weight bearing in my right leg for another six days (then it will go to 100% weight bearing as tolerated – or regular walking – Praise God!). I didn't put all my weight on my right leg today, but I was able to do my regular leg exercises more efficiently – higher leg lifts, and even as I lifted it to the back it went up a little higher more easily.

The other awesome thing that happened today was I went to my church for the first time since before the accident! And boy did we have a Holy Ghost good time. Pastor didn't even preach... the Spirit of the Lord took over the service as we worshipped God in song and prophetic words and healing touches all throughout the entire service.

I can't tell you how many times I got on my knees at my chair to worship God in tears. And to think when I first had my accident I couldn't even kneel down because of the pain. I couldn't even go to the restroom on my own without calling a nurse first. But now I can have my caregiver take me to church and with the assistance of my rolling walker with a seat (love that thing, it's so multifunctional) I could stand up and get my praise on while holding onto the handle, and I can turn around and kneel down on my knees and worship my Heavenly Father with no assistance. To God be all the Glory! He is so faithful and He loves me so much. This ordeal has definitely drawn me closer to Him. Though I questioned Him before, I dare not question Him now. He has shown Himself strong in me time and time again, His faithfulness outweighs any doubts. There is nothing my little puny mind can conceive that my God hasn't already figured out. He knows the end from the beginning. He saw me healed and praising and worshipping Him again before I did. He never doubted so why should I? Or why did I?

I thank God for His grace and forgiveness, for forgiving me for relying on my own frail strength and inferior wisdom to try and predict the outcome and doom me to anything less than total victory.

So for what I've learned, I want to commit the same challenge to you.

I want to challenge you to trust God even when you don't see the outcome.

Trust God even in those dark, broken places in your life where all you see is gloom and doom and all you feel is pain.

Trust God when you can't see how your ends will be met, where your next meal is coming from, where the next job will be or what your next business decision or relationship decision will be.

Trust God when you need a healing or a breakthrough.

Trust God that not only will He do it, but that He will do it for you.

God can, and He will, for you.

He loves you so much, He simply just wants you to trust Him with your hopes, give him all your fears and cast all of your cares on Him. Why? Because He cares for you.

Scripture says in *1 Peter 5:7* in the Amplified Version of the Bible:

Casting the whole of your care [all your anxieties, all your worries, all your concerns, once and for all] on Him, for He cares for you affectionately and cares about you watchfully.

So go ahead and cast, or throw all of your anxieties, worries and concerns once and for all on God.

Just like if you were in a baseball game and you were about to pitch…throw that ball of worry, fear and concern to the Lord, the first person who should come to your mind and the first person at bat, and as you throw those things to Him once and for all watch Him take your worries, fears and anxieties and lead them to your victory as He hits a home run in your life.

The blessed part about casting your care on Him is once you give your worries and concerns over to Him, you no longer have to think about it.

Just like after the accident, though my flesh went through its pity parties on different occasions, I eventually had to learn to surrender all and cast my worries and cares on Him.

As I rest I have to believe I also heal.

With every physical therapy session I have to believe it's getting me one step closer to my healing and full and complete recovery. With every step I take I have to believe that one day, real soon, I will walk on my own again. But first it must start with my casting that care on the Lord.

I can't believe something will happen for me if I don't first believe that God will do it. I can't believe He's going to heal me if I don't first believe He already has.

Each step I take with my walker is one step closer to my true destiny of walking again.

I literally have to walk by faith and not by sight.

Though by sight, I read about stories where legs didn't heal properly after fractures and I read about one leg being shorter than the other and I read about horror stories of people not being able to walk properly again, but I have to dismiss those "sight" claims, or bad reports, and walk by faith.

Sure "they say" it could take up to two years for me to totally heal, but I can't believe what they say, which in most cases is often the worst case scenario. I have to believe, instead, what God says.

I have to believe Him when He says in 1 Peter 2:24:

Who his own self bare our sins in his own body on the tree, that we, being dead to sins, should live unto righteousness: by whose stripes ye were healed.

I have to believe that when Jesus died on the cross for my sins over 2,000 years ago that not only was it for my sins but also for my healing and that by His stripes I am healed right now – before I see the victory. With walker in tow I have to see the light at the end of the tunnel, before it even appears. And you have to do the same.

No matter what situation you may be going through right now, you have to see the victory in advance right now and you have to cast every last one of your cares on Him because He cares for you affectionately and watchfully.

God always watches over you, and He will never leave you alone.

CHAPTER 13
THE PROCESS

Friday, May 29

Today's the big day! What day is that?

It's full-weight bearing Friday!

I was so excited all day today because, according to my surgeon, this is the day where I can put full weight on my right, fractured leg.

I walked into physical therapy today like a kid on Christmas morning, excited because I waited so long for this very moment. You see, for the first seven weeks since the accident I was only at zero percent weight bearing, meaning I couldn't put any weight on my right leg – all weight had to be put on my left leg. I remember during my hospital stay I named both my legs; my left leg was named Gordon (for "Good Leg") and my right leg was named

Renita (for "Recovering Leg"). For most of the time Gordon pretty much took care of his little sister, Renita, with everything, but with my now being full weight bearing, it's time for Renita to grow up.

The interesting thing, though, is during physical therapy I was surprised that as I was given new exercises to try as a result of my new weight bearing status, my right leg often couldn't cooperate on her own. As I did the up the stairs/down the stairs exercise with a few steps, Renita would shake uncontrollably like a leaf to the point that the physical therapist had to hold her during many of the exercises.

I couldn't understand what was going on, but my therapist explained that my right leg is like a baby learning to walk again for the first time. Since I hadn't put any pressure on that leg in so long, it was still weak and would shake as a result of lacking strength. He explained that eventually it will regain strength, but in the meantime I had to continue with exercises so it can get 100 percent back to normal.

This discovery amazed me and made me think about how healing is often a process.

Many times we want the instant blessing or the instant manifestation, without realizing that the healing took place the moment you asked God to heal you, and so now that you've asked, the time between the last prayer you prayed and the manifestation of total and complete healing is called the process. Some processes may take longer than others, but the healing has still taken place just the same.

There were many cases where people were healed in the Bible. Some instantaneously, some not.

This reminds me of the Word of God when Jesus healed the ten lepers and the Bible describes how they were healed "as they went":

> *And as he entered into a certain village, there met him ten men that were lepers, which stood afar off:*
> *And they lifted up their voices, and said, Jesus, Master, have mercy on us.*
> *And when he saw them, he said unto them, Go shew yourselves unto the priests. And it came to pass, that, as they went, they were cleansed. Luke 17:12-14*

In this example, the ten lepers were healed once Jesus declared healing in their lives, however the manifestation took place as they went. So from the time they were prayed for by Jesus to the manifestation of the healing was the process.

The same way that though my femur was broken in three places, the moment I prayed to God for Him to heal it, and the process of going through therapy and more, all this is necessary in order for the healing to take place, I just have to know and believe that it will fully take place.

In the same manner whatever it is you may be going through that needs healing, whether physically, emotionally or whatever your specific situation, it's simply a mater of trusting God throughout the entire process.

Even though the process may seem a bit shaky and weak, don't go by what's going on right now on the outside, go by the promise God made to you on the inside.

As I go through physical therapy, though I was saddened at my shaking leg, I know the more I continue to show up for therapy and do what they tell me to do, the more I will eventually be healed totally and completely.

Same thing for you – whatever you're going through, keep showing up to God in prayer and do what He tells you to do, and victory will surely be waiting for you on the other side.

CHAPTER 14
FROM GLORY TO GLORY

Tuesday, June 7

G ood morning, Jesus.

I could feel I woke up today and I could feel it – another notch of healing kicked in.

Another victory took place in my leg last night just like the time before.

I know the surgeon will confirm it – just like he did last time.
It's my testimony for today.

And now that I think more about it, that's what testimonies are – reminders of God's goodness.

It's amazing how you can feel a testimony come on before it even happens. That's what faith is. But in my case God confirmed His healing in me regarding my recovery. Not only that, because I experienced it before, I know it happened, because He did it before and He'll do it again. That's what testimonies are.

When you think about your life and what God delivered you from, you may be experiencing something that may be all too familiar.

You may be going through something that you battled before.

That same demon may have showed up before, but remember just like you beat him before you will do it again.

Just like God delivered you before, He will deliver you again.

Be sure and remember your past testimonies and use that to fuel your faith when faced with opposition yet again.

Remember that Jesus is the same yesterday, today and forever (Hebrews 13:8) and if He did it for you before . . . (you fill in the rest ☺). If He healed you before, He will heal you again. In broken places, remember who you are and whose you are and that all the promises of God for you are still yes and amen.

Why?

Because He is an amazing God and He loves you.

The LORD hath appeared of old unto me, saying, Yea, I have loved thee with an everlasting love: therefore with lovingkindness have I drawn thee. Jeremiah 31:3

CHAPTER 15
DON'T LOOK BACK

Sunday, June 21

So today, as I went to open the door for my caregiver this morning I, out of a previous habit, grabbed my rolling walker. Once I grabbed it, I walked slower than I had in a long time, and it appeared as if my whole countenance changed into dismal and gloomy. What at first seemed like a good morning suddenly, upon grabbing the rolling walker, turned into a weak reminder of pain.

Once I opened the door I realized that I had grabbed the walker by mistake.

I was supposed to grab my cane, as I had recently, since May 29, graduated from my walker to a cane. So far I literally have gone from being in a wheelchair to a walker to a cane, but for some reason on this particular day I totally forgot about my graduation and reverted back to the past.

And once I grabbed hold of the past, my spirit left with it.

Sometimes in life, as God would have us in progression mode, we somehow still want to hold onto something from the past that not only reminds us of a dark place but also crushes our souls and weakens our spirits.

God always wants us to move forward.

We're the ones who often, sometimes even unknowingly, get stuck in the past.

Just like Lot's wife in the book of Genesis, as God led them out of Sodom so they wouldn't be destroyed with everyone else, the one thing that she was asked to do in order to make it safely to the other side was to not look back.

As she pressed ahead with her husband, instead of continuing to go in the direction of victory, she made the conscious decision to turn around and look back. And what was the result of her looking back? She was turned into a pillar of salt, and never made it to her very own promised land.

She never made it to her safe place.

She never reached her destiny.

She died before she realized victory was waiting for her on the other side of her obedience. If only she didn't look back *(Genesis 19:24-26).*

As the Lord blesses us progressively we must remember to not look back.

We must remember to leave the past in the past, and not take a hold of things from the past that cause us to move backward instead of forward.

As we walk by faith and run this Christian race, we must continue to press ahead not only the way we are, but the way we're meant to be.

Which reminds me of someone else from the Bible, Bartimaeus.

Before coming to Jesus, Bartimaeus was a blind beggar. But as soon as he heard Jesus was nearby, he ran toward Jesus, throwing off his beggar's clothes, and yelled, "Jesus! Thou son of David! Have mercy on me!" *(Mark 10:47)*

The word, *mercy*, in this Scripture means not only have mercy on, but it also means to help the afflicted or help one seeking aid. So, in essence Bartimaeus was crying out, "Jesus! Help me!"

But notice that not only did he cry out, as he got closer to Jesus in the crowd. The Scripture describes how he threw off his old clothes:

> *And when he heard that it was Jesus of Nazareth, he began to cry out, and say, Jesus, thou son of David, have mercy on me.*
>
> *And many charged him that he should hold his peace: but he cried the more a great deal, Thou son of David, have mercy on me.*
>
> *And Jesus stood still, and commanded him to be called. And they call the blind man, saying unto him, Be of good comfort, rise; he calleth thee.*
>
> *And he, casting away his garment, rose, and came to Jesus.*
>
> *Mark 10:47-50*

Though the crowd initially told him to be quiet, because Bartimaeus knew what he needed and what he wanted, he ignored them and cried even louder. And as soon as he was told that Jesus beckoned him to come forth, he, knowing what that meant, cast away his garment, or threw away his old clothes.

Bartimaeus knew his old clothes represented where he was, as a blind beggar, and that by casting them off, it was representing where he was going, which was to Jesus – the Healer!

And Jesus answered and said unto him, What wilt thou that I should do unto thee? The blind man said unto him, Lord, that I might receive my sight.
And Jesus said unto him, Go thy way; thy faith hath made thee whole. And immediately he received his sight, and followed Jesus in the way. Mark 10:51-52

And as a result of Bartimaeus going after Jesus and shedding himself of the past, not only was he healed he was also made whole!

So though it may have seemed like a frivolous mistake, I pledge never to grab hold of that ole rolling walker ever again, because since then I have called on Jesus and since then He is the one making me whole and I can't turn back; I won't turn back and neither should you – ever again.

Brethren, I count not myself to have apprehended: but this one thing I do, forgetting those things which are behind, and reaching forth unto those things which are before,
I press toward the mark for the prize of the high calling of God in Christ Jesus. Philippians 3:13-14

CHAPTER 16

THE POWER OF COMMUNITY

Wednesday, June 24

Today I had a good day at physical therapy.

Now in week seven of outpatient physical therapy, I got my workout on, consisting of walking on the elliptical machine (at speed of 2.0; hey, gotta start somewhere…Despise not small beginnings lol), stretching with the rubber band thingy wrapped around my leg, lying against the large round ball on the wall and going up and down to strengthen my leg muscles, using the three steps for strengthening and balance, and lastly my two favorites which include my fifteen-minute cooldown where they place a heating pack on my leg. I literally use this time to meditate. And the stretching time where the therapist would stretch my leg out and challenge me to use it in ways I never had before.

Though, admittedly, I look forward to a good workout every time, the best part about physical therapy, for me, is the community.

Every time I enter the gym room I am greeted with "Hello, Kim" and warm smiles from the four-man staff consisting of Roger, Richard, Ryan and the manager, Ed. (All R's and an E? Weird, I know lol.) I take that back, when I first come in I'm greeted with a warm and loving "Hi, Kim!" from the desk receptionist, April, who keeps me abreast of the latest hair trends and best deals on her cute summer wardrobe buys. THEN the guys speak once I enter the gym, and not only that, my fellow "trainers" as I like to call them, as they train in order to get well day by day, like me, speak to me as well. We all are there as a result of injury from car accidents, and we all want to be well, but it's refreshing to be in a loving, supportive environment where you don't always know what to expect – whether it's the older lady with the kinky mouth, the young lady explaining the details of her latest real estate deal, the conversation of the day about relationships and how, as Richard often states, men and women can *never* be just friends (I beg to differ lol), or whether it's the latest joke from the older lady that no one ever seems to get, but all seem to appreciate anyway.

It's important, with whatever you're going through, that you surround yourself with a positive, supportive environment.

A wise minister once said, go where you're celebrated, and not simply tolerated.

Even Jesus, as He ministered to the masses, also retreated to the home of His friends and inner circle such as to

Martha, Mary and Lazarus' house, or even Peter's house for dinner as He healed Peter's mother-in-law who, once healed, served them all afterward. *(Matthew 8:14-15)*

Jesus retreated to a place where others knew His name and where He felt comfortable.

He wasn't just an island or a preaching machine all by Himself.

Even during those mornings when He had His alone time to pray, He still always made time to interact and heal not only the masses but spend quality time with His true friends.

Know that whatever you're going through, you're not alone – so don't be alone.

Find the blessing in your community and allow other people to help and assist you if you need help.

I know, for me, when I was in the hospital and soon after I came out and was on my walker, the Lord blessed me with tons of visits from my spiritual and physical family who brought food and other items just to bless me. As a normally independent person who's used to doing things on my own, I had to get used to other people wanting to take care of me. I had to realize that, for some, it actually blessed them to be able to be a blessing to me. I had to find the blessing in my community, and once I did I had to embrace and simply say "Thank you, Jesus" for those whom He had brought in my life to be a blessing.

Then shall the King say unto them on his right hand, Come, ye blessed of my Father, inherit the kingdom prepared for you from the foundation of the world:

For I was an hungred, and ye gave me meat: I was thirsty, and ye gave me drink: I was a stranger, and ye took me in:

Naked, and ye clothed me: I was sick, and ye visited me: I was in prison, and ye came unto me. Matthew 25:34-36

CHAPTER 17

PREPARING TO FACE THE GIANTS AGAIN

Saturday, June 26

So today I took the ultimate leap of faith since the accident tragedy that broke my right femur. Since my car was totaled in the accident, I went out today, three months since the accident, and I bought another one.

What normally was a common daily commute for most people now became a frightening activity that, as I experienced, could lead to a two-week stay in a dark, lonely hospital room.

What was once a habitual thing to do on a once friendly road became a tumultuous journey in a land of impatient strangers behind the wheel of more than 5,000-pound missiles that seem to be aimed right at me.

What used to be mere innocent drivers are now giants to me and I seem small, as the car accident I experienced reduced me to a small state of helplessness.

I must believe the roads love me.

I must believe the roads support me and are on my side.

I must find a car I like, test drive it and buy. I must get behind the wheel again with confidence. It's the only way I can face those giants again in order to remain sane.

And eventually, I did.

You may be facing your own giant – which may have returned.

It could have been cancer remission – where you thought the cancer was gone as pronounced by your doctor as you and your family praised and thanked God, but it may have come back again, even more fierce this time as it may have spread. You still have to continue to believe that God is still a Healer, and that He can heal you – no matter how big the giant you may face.

Don't see yourself as small compared to a giant circumstance. See yourself as BIG.

In the Bible, when David faced the giant, Goliath, David didn't see himself as small. He saw himself as big. He saw himself as a conqueror. He saw himself as a victor, before the fight even began.

> *Then said David to the Philistine, Thou comest to me with a sword, and with a spear, and with a shield: but I come to thee in the name of the LORD of hosts, the God of the armies of Israel, whom though hast defied.*
>
> *This day will the LORD deliver thee into mine hand; and I will smite thee, and take thine head from thee; and I will give the carcasses of the host of the Philistines this day*

unto the fowls of the air, and to the beasts of the earth; that
all the earth may know that there is a God in Israel.
And all this assembly shall know that the LORD saveth
not with sword and spear: for the battle is the LORD's, and
he will give you into our hands. 1 Samuel 17:45-47

David, a shepherd boy, was so confident that he would win
while facing his giant that he even insisted on fighting
Goliath in spite of others' objections.

And Saul said to David, Thou art not able to go against
this Philistine to fight with him: for thou art but a youth,
and he a man of war from his youth. 1 Samuel 17:33

But instead of agreeing with the naysayer, David decided to
put Saul in his place by reminding him (and himself) of his
previous victories:

And David said unto Saul, Thy servant kept his father's
sheep, and there came a lion, and a bear, and took a lamb
out of the flock:
And I went out after him, and smote him, and deliv-
ered it out of his mouth: and when he arose against me, I
caught him by his beard, and smote him, and slew him.
Thy servant slew both the lion and the bear: and this
uncircumcised Philistine shall be as one of them, seeing he
hath defied the armies of the living God.
David said moreover, The LORD that delivered me out
of the paw of the lion, and out of the paw of the bear, he

*will deliver me out of the hand of this Philistine. And Saul
said unto David, Go, and the LORD be with thee. 1 Samuel
17:34-37*

Here, David was able to turn his initial doubter, Saul, into
a believer.

David's confidence in His God and his past victories
caused others to have faith in him as well.

In the same manner, your confidence in the God you
serve and your past victories and testimonies will build the
confidence of those around you as well.

When facing new giants, remember how God delivered
you from an old giant, and don't be afraid to face it again
with more confidence for a bigger challenge.

David's first challenge was small, now this one with
Goliath was big.

Sometimes overcoming smaller obstacles in life is God's
preparation for us to face and defeat bigger giants.

Have faith in the God that delivered you then, and He'll
deliver you now.

David faced his giant head on and won. His victory was
not only for himself (as his reward was riches, the king's
daughter's hand and freedom for his family, *1 Samuel 17:25*)
but it also freed the land and delivered them from the fear
of being overthrown by a monstrous giant.

Remember that, as you face your giant head on, your
victory will not be just for you but also for the thousands
of people who will be blessed by your testimony that will
inspire them to face their giants as well.

Your restoration and recovery will restore and recover
someone else (the same way, I pray, my restoration and

recovery is restoring and recovering you). God's will is always that we, His children, go from glory to glory in every circumstance and situation and that we edify one another while always provoking one another unto good works *(2 Corinthians 3:18, 1 Thessalonians 5:11, Hebrews 10:24)*.

We are still overcome by the blood of the Lamb and the word of our testimonies.

> *And they overcame him by the blood of the Lamb, and by the word of their testimony; and they loved not their lives unto the death. Revelations 12:11*

The word, *overcame,* in this passage of Scripture in the original Greek means, to conquer, to come off victorious, and pertaining to Christians that hold fast their faith even unto death against the power of their foes, and temptations and persecutions.

Know that as you overcome, others will see your faith, strength and confidence in your God, which will cause them to want to press on and overcome and face their giants again as well.

So while I face my giant and get behind a wheel and drive again, I keep an eye on the big picture, knowing that facing this giant will actually allow me to now "go forth" to and fro to minister the Word, touch and save lives while ministering and being ministered to and ultimately blessing others.

So don't be afraid to face your giants.

Don't see yourself like the Children of Israel, who saw themselves as grasshoppers in the sight of the giants who initially inhabited their promised land *(Numbers 13:33)*. See yourself as big because you serve a big God.

See yourself as big because you serve a God who is on your side.

See yourself as more than a conqueror because you really are.

Nay, in all these things we are more than conquerors through him that loved us. Romans 8:37

Face your giants, speak the victory in advance and walk in it, or in my case, drive off into the sunset with your new ride with a renewed praise on your lips.

But I will hope continually, and will yet praise thee more and more. Psalm 71:14

CHAPTER 18

THIS IS THE DAY (NO LONGER A VICTIM)

Wednesday, July 15

Super excited about today.

This is the day I decided to no longer be a victim.

No matter what I've gone through and no matter how I may feel on any given day (pain or no pain) this is the day I decide to be free, to be whole, to be healed and to *not* be a victim.

While driving today, as I'm getting used to driving even more while no longer being afraid, I made the decision to no longer be a victim. And quite honestly, I've grown tired of the "awww" and "poor you" responses once I tell someone that I was involved in a car accident a few months ago in which my femur bone was broken. Thankfully I'm not using my cane that much, so on days I don't use it, no one has any idea that I was involved in any kind of accident. I prefer it that way. The only ones who are even made aware of the pain I went through are the ones I volunteer the information to. So today I serve notice to my past and I say, "No more!" No longer will I be a victim, as far as I'm concerned it never happened. Yup, I said it, it *never* happened.

My proclamation today reminds me of a passage of Scripture in which the Apostle Paul is accused of being a Christian killer and rabble rouser because of his past. Paul's response? He acted as if he didn't have a clue about what they were talking about *(2 Corinthians 7:2)*. The reason he does this so adamantly is because he proclaims how he forgets the past to the point of not even remembering it anymore as he states in *Philippians 3:13:*

> *Brethren, I count not myself to have apprehended: but this one thing I do, forgetting those things which are behind, and reaching forth unto those things which are before,*

So as he forgets the past, which is behind him, he reaches forth toward things that are before.

Besides, I have too many dreams yet to be realized to be stuck in the past.

I have too much to do for the Lord to be stuck in a "woe is me" state or "why did this happen to me?" frame of mind.

I have too many lives to touch, too many souls to save, too many people yet to be encouraged, entertained and inspired to be focusing on a leg that, yes, though it may get on my nerves at times, it still can move.

When I stand up, I still can walk. And, one day – real soon, I'll be able to run again.

But until then, I may not be able to run again physically (yet) I can still run my race. I can run my race in the Lord, or as my cousin, Veda, says, I can run my race with God's grace. Or as my uncle, Minister Eugene Brooks says, I can keep the faith, I can stay the course, I can enjoy the ride.

So while I'm running ahead, I can't be stuck in the pain from behind. So as a result, I denounce it.

I forget about it.

I act like it never happened, and I press ahead.

Not only that, but I propose you take the same stance as well.

No matter what you may have gone through.

No matter what storm or circumstance you may have faced.

Choose not to be the victim. Choose to be victorious!

Choose to walk in your future instead of wallowing in the past.

Don't allow people to keep you away from where God is taking you.

Only keep those in your ear who propel you into who you're going to be and not who you were. Only keep people in your ear who remind you of where you're going instead of feeling sorry for where you've been.

Wipe the slate clean and start all over again with a fresh start and a fresh perspective. Sure that may have happened to you, or may be happening to you right now, but it has nothing, absolutely nothing to do with who you are and where God is taking you.

But the path of the just is as the shining light, that shineth more and more unto the perfect day. Proverbs 4:18

CHAPTER 19

AFTER THE RAIN

Wednesday, July 29

I am so excited today! Want to know why? It's raining outside, dark and gloomy, yet inside I'm beaming because it's raining and my leg's not hurting! Yay!

You know how they say, after you've had surgery, folks be like, "Well, ya know, now that you had that surgery your leg's going to hurt every time just before it rains . . . " I mean, I've even had supposedly well-meaning Christians tell me this. When folk insist on telling me how I'm doomed to experience pain every time it rains, I simply correct them in words in order to rebuke the negative suggestion from the atmosphere and just leave the area.

Days after someone declared I was bound to experience pain every time it rained, my leg started hurting. It got to a point where it started hurting daily, especially just before it rained. Every time it did I thought about that person's words, and was actually upset that my ears heard them, because I'm like a sponge when it comes to hearing things, and I felt like subconsciously I had received what she was speaking over me. And she wasn't the only one speaking negative things over me. Other people would make comments about my having arthritis and all kinds of stuff. All the while I'm thinking to myself, "Why am I even listening to this person? Why is this person even in my space close enough to be speaking ill will over me?" Needless to say I've limited my contact with that person, and since then I have started listening to more positive, inspiring messages regularly like motivational speaker Wayne Dyer and of course my mentor, Mr. Art Cartwright, who always shares a timely Word and inspiring message.

He often speaks of the importance of environment and getting around the right people who can speak a word in due season in order to advance you, and getting away from the doubters, the nay-sayers and the haters. I believe some people are haters and they, themselves, don't even know it. Around you they present themselves as supporters and friends but then what comes out of their mouth is an entirely different story.

So, again, I've learned to limit contact with those kinds of people, and hear inspiring messages, and speak, out loud, what I want to see happen. As Scripture says, We walk by faith and not by sight, right *(2 Corinthians 5:7)* and I'm the healed and not the sick by His stripes so no, it's not a medical reality or proclamation, it's a truthful proclamation and the truth will make me free.

I was definitely freed today, right now while looking out my window at the rain pouring down.

I just returned from physical therapy about an hour ago (great session, by the way) and I didn't feel an ounce of pain before the rain, or an ounce of pain after the rain. Glo-reh!

God is so Good!

So I just want to encourage you in that whatever you're going through, surround yourself with people who will speak the Word over you and leave their own feelings, or statistics aside and simply trust God from the words coming out of their lips, which should line up with God's words.

Don't let worry or doubt creep in by way of allowing someone to speak ill over you, stay prayed up and faith-filled by hearing and hearing and hearing the Word of God. Remember, it's only Christ's words that will last. All else will only pass away. And His Word is the only healing balm you really need anyway.

> *So then faith cometh by hearing, and hearing by the word of God. Romans 10:17*
>
> *Heaven and earth shall pass away, but my words shall not pass away. Matthew 24:35*
>
> *Who his own self bare our sins in his own body on the tree, that we, being dead to sins, should live unto righteousness: by whose stripes ye were healed. 1 Peter 2:24*

CHAPTER 20
FLASHBACKS

Wednesday, August 5

So this morning I got in the shower and, for some reason, had a flashback.

I flashed back to the week I was in the hospital following the car accident. One day back then after taking a shower, while I was being escorted back to the bed by the nurse, I blanked out and woke up in bed with four or five people hovering over me. Evidently I had passed out because I had gotten too warm while in the restroom and during my hospital stay my blood count was extremely low. It's fine now, thank God, but back then it wasn't and I couldn't handle the heat in the restroom.

That was such a scary time, back then, and I was almost upset I had this flashback five months later, where I am now able to take a shower with no assistance and no bath chair – to God be the glory!

Sometimes, while driving, I flash back to the car accident and I see the other driver shoot out of the side street, ignoring the stop sign, as I swerved to avoid him but it was too late. I hate those flashbacks. When I have them I have to remember to cast them down in Jesus' Name because Lord knows I don't want that to happen again. I wouldn't wish what happened to me on my worst enemy.

You may have gone through something in the past, something horrific like an accident, a beating by a loved one, a traumatic hospital experience or death of a loved one or something like that, and often you, too, may flash back to dark moments.

Well, I'd like to encourage you to do what I've learned to do during those times, cast them down.

Cast down those thoughts and imaginations that are not of God.

Don't allow the enemy access to your mind, and definitely don't let him control your mind.

It's the devil who wants us to remain stuck in the past while reminding us of the past, while it's always God who wants us to continue to press ahead and move forward.

Thoughts from the past are to be bound and cast out in Jesus' Name. Only then will you receive freedom and victory, and who the son sets free is free indeed.

Casting down imaginations, and every high thing that exalteth itself against the knowledge of God, and bringing into captivity every thought to the obedience of Christ; 2 Corinthians 10:5

Verily I say unto you, Whatsoever ye shall bind on earth shall be bound in heaven: and whatsoever ye shall loose on earth shall be loosed in heaven. Matthew 18:18

CHAPTER 21
DON'T DO IT!

Friday, August 7

Today while driving I had a moment to think about some things in my life I wasn't quite happy about. I know I hadn't mentioned this before, but right now my mother is having some serious health challenges. I, and others, have prayed for her and I know she's healed in Jesus' name, but some days I just want *her* to know she's healed. Meantime, I have to have enough faith for both of us, but this particular day, after delivering her breakfast as is custom, I started to feel bad about what she's been going through, what I have been going through, and I was this close to crying but then the following words came out of my mouth, *"Don't do it!"*

Immediately after I said those three words out loud, the tears which were about to fall dried up before they even had a chance to touch skin.

Next thing you know I kept saying it, *"Don't do it! Don't do it! Don't do it!"* over and over again.

I found myself regaining more and more strength each time I said it.

There is power in words, more importantly though, there is power in our words when we speak God's will over our lives.

God doesn't want us to "go there" with our emotions, so I didn't want to either.

God didn't want me to "do it," "it" meaning have a pity party because of the storms I'm facing right now. Though as tempting as it is some days, those three words remind me that I will not "go" where the enemy wants me to "go" which is to a place of pain emotionally and a world of sadness.

Instead, God wants to restore the joy I once had. He wants to even restore the joy I had when I first got saved, when I was seeking His face daily, early in the morning an hour a day, serving Him most of the week, praying for people all the time and loving it – He wants to restore that back. And there's no way He can restore all that back and take back what the devil stole from me if I lie somewhere crying over spilled milk.

So, no, I won't go there, and I want to encourage you not to go there either.

Next time the enemy throws a negative thought in your mind or the next time you feel your back is against the wall and that your troubles are too much, remember God will not allow you to handle more than you can bear and that you have mountain-moving power on the inside of you.

So not only should you cast down imaginations and negative thoughts when they come, but also speak over yourself, like one of my favorite songs says, and remind the devil who's in charge.

"Don't do it!"

For verily I say unto you, That whosoever shall say unto this mountain, Be thou removed, and be thou cast into the sea; and shall not doubt in his heart, but shall believe that those things which he saith shall come to pass; he shall have whatsoever he saith. Mark 11:23

There hath no temptation taken you but such as is common to man: but God is faithful, who will not suffer you to be tempted above that ye are able; but will with the temptation also make a way to escape, that ye may be able to bear it. 1 Corinthians 10:13

Come unto me, all ye that labour and are heavy laden, and I will give you rest. Take my yoke upon you, and learn of me; for I am meek and lowly in heart: and ye shall find rest unto your souls. For my yoke is easy, and my burden is light. Matthew 11:28-30

CHAPTER 22
WHOSE REPORT WILL I BELIEVE?

Saturday, August 15

Unfortunately the other day I got some bad news from the doctor.

Just when I thought this eBook was almost finished I got some news from my rehab doctor concerning the bone that's been growing inside my leg. She said I developed something called heterotopic ossification, which basically means I've grown more bone inside my leg than I'm supposed to. Bone is growing outside of the confines of where it should be. It's not a large amount, but enough for the X-ray to catch it. It's something that normally occurs in the case of one who has had a hip replacement surgery, and I guess the surgery I had was similar. No wonder I have this small patch of extra fat that appears on my hip. At first my physical therapist thought it was just fluid, but now it looks like it's from the inflammation as a result of this condition. I hate satan!

Honestly, when the doctor told me the news a couple days ago on Thursday I immediately grew sad and disappointed.

I felt like I thought I was doing so well.

Now I felt like this was a setback.

However as soon as I prayed to God about it He reminded me in a Scripture study I'm currently doing. Recently I decided to read the entire Bible over from the very beginning in Genesis. I'm now in Exodus, on the story of Moses where he was challenged as the chosen one to demand that the Egyptian king Pharoah let his people, the Hebrew people aka the children of Israel, go.

When God chose Moses to do the job, Moses hesitated.

He came up with every excuse why he shouldn't be the chosen one. He even mentioned how his speech wasn't eloquent, and God even worked with Moses and told him that his brother, Aaron, would speak for him.

God challenged Moses to step up to Pharoah, and God even warned Moses that at first Pharoah would not immediately let his people go because his heart would be hardened and God wanted to show forth His miracles to the children of Israel so that they would know that it was God who delivered them and not Moses and definitely not they themselves.

Well, when Moses first went to tell the children of Israel that he was the chosen sent one by God sent to deliver them from slavery, the Egyptian slave master's response was to make it harder for them to work, punishing and beating them. This made the children of Israel furious with Moses.

They felt since Moses' arrival and proclamations of future freedom things only grew worse.

Even Moses complained to God when he states, *For since I came to Pharaoh to speak in thy name, he hath done evil to this people; neither hast thou delivered thy people at all. Exodus 5:23*

Moses' response was to accuse God.

Because Moses didn't see the results God promised immediately and because the situation got worse than better, Moses assumed God did not keep His word.

Moses saw an outcome of failure based on the present circumstance when God saw an outcome of victory.

God knew the children of Israel would be delivered – by the hand of Moses.

He knew Pharoah's heart would eventually soften to let them go, but Moses had to believe it, too, and he was having trouble believing, because he wasn't "seeing."

God used this Scripture to remind me, in my current situation, though it felt like victory was around the corner and then it suddenly turned worse by way of a bad report, that doesn't mean God doesn't hold the final outcome to my own personal victory.

Just because the doctor said I have extra bone growing out of my leg, doesn't mean I have to believe her report.

I chose to believe the report of the Lord, and God says I'm HEALED!

God says, I'm DELIVERED!

God says I shall LIVE and NOT DIE, and I will declare the works of the Lord.

What I'm going through SHALL BE a testimony to all who are going through something right now.

That no matter what you're going through . . . God holds the outcome!

He sees the ending from the beginning.

Just because you may see giants in the land, God still said to go and take it, because He already planned to take care of those giants.

He just wants us to trust Him, and His Word, and move forward and do whatever He has called us to do.

So no, I will not have a pity party.

I will hold my head up high and walk out the victory God has called me to.

I bind satan in Jesus' name, I proclaim (as I lay hands on my leg) that my leg is healed, and whole in the name of Jesus!

There's no extra bone, it will shrivel up and shrink right now, and there is just the right amount of bone that I need for total and complete healing! – In Jesus' Name!

It IS so.

And these signs shall follow them that believe; In my name shall they cast out devils; they shall speak with new tongues;

They shall take up serpents; and if they drink any deadly thing, it shall not hurt them; they shall lay hands on the sick, and they shall recover. Mark 16:17-18

CHAPTER 23
I FORGOT

Thursday, August 20

Tonight I attended Bible study at Global Empowerment and the Word was so good I was praising God on the inside, and afterward a young lady came up to me and leaped for joy when she saw me. I'm normally friendly with everyone but this one particular person tickled me because she was so happy to see me that I felt like I was Mary from the Bible when Sarah saw her and she said her baby, John, leapt for joy on the inside at the sound of Mary's voice *(Luke 1:41)*.

I just attributed it to the God in me, but then she went on to say, "Kim! I'm so happy to see you because I thought about what was shared on the prayer call last week and how you said the doctors complimented you on how fast your recovery was taking place and how they initially said it would take over a year for you to recover!"

Bless her heart. God is good, and her words definitely reminded me of God's faithfulness, but they also reminded me of something else . . . the accident, the injury, the broken femur...all of which I had totally forgotten about prior to our conversation!

And I shared that with her. I shared how God is SO GOOD in that until she brought it up, at that moment, following Bible study, I had totally forgotten about my previous pain.

The anointing of God was so strong, that for that brief moment, it was as if I was totally normal and just like the accident NEVER HAPPENED.

Glory be to God.

God is so faithful, in that no matter what you may be going through right now, He will restore you to your previous position of wholeness, your previous position of peace and your previous position of thankfulness in that you won't even feel like what you have been through!

Just like with our sins, when we repent and ask Him for forgiveness, once we call on Jesus' Name, confess and petition the blood of Jesus, God restores us right back to right standing with Him. Once again we are whole, pure and complete in His sight, as if we never sinned in the first place.

God is a healer, and a restorer.

He will heal you, He will restore you and He will cause you to remember the pain no more.

And I will restore to you the years that the locust hath eaten, the cankerworm, and the caterpiller, and the palmerworm, my great army which I sent among you. Joel 2:25

Come now, and let us reason together, saith the LORD: *though your sins be as scarlet, they shall be as white as snow; though they be red like crimson, they shall be as wool. Isaiah 1:18*

Therefore if any man be in Christ, he is a new creature: old things are passed away; behold, all things are become new. 2 Corinthians 5:17

If we confess our sins, he is faithful and just to forgive us our sins and to cleanse us from all unrighteousness. 1 John 1:9

CHAPTER 24

TEMPTATION IN THE WILDERNESS

Friday, August 21

So I just completed my first week at a new physical therapy office.

Though I loved the last office, I had to go with a different one because the first one has a policy where after twelve weeks they want you to continue from home for six weeks before starting again. Well, my doctor didn't think that would be a good idea since I was progressing so nicely so my case manager found me a new physical therapy location.

This one is turning out to be okay so far. I was a little miffed because the first day I had to wait an hour after my appointment before I was seen and then the second day one of their vans was down so they were an hour late in picking me up and once there I had to wait another 30 minutes after signing in before starting. At the other physical therapy location there was no waiting whatsoever. You just signed in and headed straight back to the gym area to work out. Well, I mentioned my unhappiness, thus far, to the new manager (I had actually Googled a newer location because I was ready to switch) and he turned out to be very accommodating by stating once I sign in I can head straight back to workout like I was accustomed to, then the other massage type therapy can all be done last. Also, the staff up front were very apologetic about the tardiness and they remained polite and professional the whole time so ultimately I decided to go ahead and give this new place a chance. So after the first two days, on today's visit (the last for the week since I attend three days a week) I was told by the physical therapist that my right leg was still weak from the accident and because I haven't been using the muscles that much from it since I was deferring to using the other, better leg mostly. For example, when I walk without the cane I may lean over to the right side, mainly because I can feel the added pressure to my right leg, so instead of feeling that I opt to put all the weight on my left leg (Gordon). I know Gordon's the big brother and that he loves taking care of his little sister, Renita, but it's time for Gordon to let Renita spread her wings a little bit so Renita can start to fly on her own.

So my therapist suggested I use my cane if it became uncomfortable to walk regularly without it, because he didn't want me, years down the line, to walk with a limp (which makes sense as I don't want that either).

He also told me that during this next six weeks of therapy we will focus on gateway exercises (so I can walk regularly and straight effortlessly without feeling any pressure) and also building muscle in the pelvis area of my right leg which was weak. He gave me some bed exercises to do to target those muscles and some standing up exercises. Though I could feel slight pain from the pressure, since I hadn't been using those muscles as much before, I could tell the more I did it, the more the pain went away.

So now God is taking me from healing to muscle building, which may describe your walk as well.

It's important that we, as believers, though we may appear healed and okay on the outside, that we continue to build up our faith muscles by remaining in the Word so we can remain strengthened daily on the inside.

Don't let the devil catch you slipping at a moment of weakness.

It's important to build those faith muscles up now so that when the tempter comes (and he will) you won't fall into a ditch and be led astray.

Just like when satan tempted Jesus.

Satan tempted Jesus in the wilderness with charging him to turn the stone to be made bread especially after Jesus just fasted 40 days and 40 nights. Satan knew, as a result of the fast, that Jesus was weak and hungry and he wanted to tempt Jesus by questioning His own identity because if Jesus admitted He couldn't do it then He would be telling satan that he is more powerful than Jesus is (which we know is not true).

But that's what satan does. He tempts you during weak points. But though Jesus was weak in the flesh He was strong in the Spirit in that His response was the Word of God:

But he answered and said, It is written, Man shall not live by bread alone, but by every word that proceedeth out of the mouth of God. Matthew 4:4

Satan didn't stop there. He next tempted Jesus to throw himself down from the pinnacle, or highest point of the pinnacle, in essence tempting Jesus to commit suicide. But Jesus didn't buy this trick either; again He responded with the Word of God:

Jesus said unto him, It is written again, Thou shalt not tempt the Lord thy God. Matthew 4:7

And then satan tempted Jesus a third time, this time by appealing to the pride of man (the same sin that caused both satan and Adam to fall) and told Jesus if He would only bow down and worship him, he would give Him all the kingdoms of the world *(Matthew 4:9)*. Still not impressed (and not tainted with the sin of pride as Jesus was sinless) Jesus responded, yet again, with a Word response:

Then saith Jesus unto him, Get thee hence, Satan: for it is written, Thou shalt worship the Lord thy God, and him only shalt thou serve. Matthew 4:10

So finally satan left Jesus, and the angels came and ministered to, or served Jesus after His first victory over the enemy *(Matthew 10:11)*.

Jesus won the battle because of two reasons: He remembered who He was in Christ Jesus, and He knew His God so that nothing the devil said, which was contrary to God's

Word or God's character, would be believed, because Jesus knows His Father.

I and my Father are one. John 10:30

Jesus wasn't about to let the devil shake Him. Jesus had built up his faith in God's Word so much that even at a point of weakness in the flesh after a fast, Jesus still knew to call on His help and allow God to speak through Him so that the devil would eventually have to bow down to Him or run away.

Same thing with you.

During this season, as you go through this storm (and as God has already healed and restored you) remember to keep building up your faith muscles day by day so you will be ready to strike with your sword and your shield the next time the enemy tries to attack. Remember he can try, but it's in your power to cause him not to win.

The devil's all roar and no bite; and you always get the victory in the end.

> *Be sober, be vigilant; because your adversary the devil, as a roaring lion, walketh about, seeking whom he may devour: 1 Peter 5:8*

> *But thanks be to God, which giveth us the victory through our Lord Jesus Christ. 1 Corinthians 15:57*

> *Finally, my brethren, be strong in the Lord, and in the power of his might.*
> *Put on the whole armour of God, that ye may be able to stand against the wiles of the devil.*

For we wrestle not against flesh and blood, but against principalities, against powers, against the rulers of the darkness of this world, against spiritual wickedness in high places.

Wherefore take unto you the whole armour of God, that ye may be able to withstand in the evil day, and having done all, to stand.

Stand therefore, having your loins girt about with truth, and having on the breastplate of righteousness;

And your feet shod with the preparation of the gospel of peace;

Above all, taking the shield of faith, wherewith ye shall be able to quench all the fiery darts of the wicked.

And take the helmet of salvation, and the sword of the Spirit, which is the word of God:

Praying always with all prayer and supplication in the Spirit, and watching thereunto with all perseverance and supplication for all saints;

Ephesians 6:10-18

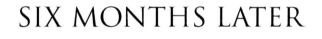

SIX MONTHS LATER

CHAPTER 25

REAL TRUST

Tuesday, September 14

Well, it's been exactly six months since the car accident.

Though I can still remember it like it was yesterday, I thank God that He has brought me from a mighty long way.

I went from surgery to having to be wheeled in a wheelchair, to using a regular walker, then a rollator walker, then a cane and now, for the most part I don't even use a cane at all unless I have to (which isn't that often). Hallelujah! To God be all the Glory!

God is so faithful, and when I think back on all He's brought me from I can only say, "Thank You." I honestly feel if He doesn't do anything else for me, I will have lived a full life, full of love and joy in Him. I now understand what the Scripture says when it speaks of joy unspeakable and full of glory *(1 Peter 1:8).* That's one thing this whole ordeal has taught me, how, when you go through something, with God on your side you're not only never alone but there is always victory on the other side. One thing about when you go through, no matter how many people pray for you or call you or express care and concern (and trust me, I appreciate all the care and expressions of love I have received even up to this point) only two people know all the pain and hurt you experienced, and that's you and God. No one else understands, but they can show that they care which is, indeed, a blessing. But even if you feel like you don't have anyone in your corner right now, or if you feel like no one cares, know that God cares, and He's all you need.

He's all you need to go through the storm, and He's all you need to make it over to the other side.

It reminds me of the story in the Bible of the prophet Elisha when he was about to be attacked by the king of Aram's army. One of Elisha's soldiers grew worried because the king's army was so large in number.

> *And when the servant of the man of God was risen early, and gone forth, behold, an host compassed the city both with horses and chariots. And his servant said unto him, Alas, my master! how shall we do?*
>
> *And he answered, Fear not: for they that be with us are more than they that be with them.*
>
> *And Elisha prayed, and said, LORD, I pray thee, open his eyes, that he may see. And the LORD opened the eyes of the young man; and he saw: and, behold, the mountain was full of horses and chariots of fire round about Elisha.*
> *2 Kings 6:15-17*

The prophet Elisha knew God was on His side and would fight his battle for him, yet he had to convince his servant of the same. So when Elisha prayed that God would open the young man's eyes so he may see all the angels ready to fight the battle, it was only then that the servant was convinced.

Sometimes, as we go through something, we tend to forget who's really on our side and the fact that God has already positioned a host of angels and other spiritual warriors to battle for you as you're going through. Even the Scripture explains how Jesus is our great mediator who also makes intercession for us.

> . . . *It is Christ that died, yea rather, that is risen again, who is even at the right hand of God, who also maketh intercession for us. Romans 8:34*

> *But to which of the angels said he at any time, Sit on my right hand, until I make thine enemies thy footstool?*
> *Are they not all ministering spirits, sent forth to minister for them who shall be heirs of salvation? Hebrews 1:13-14*

> *And there appeared an angel unto him from heaven, strengthening him. Luke 22:43*

So as you go through, not only do you have God on your side, you have his angels ministering to you, strengthening you and also fighting for you, and you have Jesus praying for you.

As you go through, pay special attention to the people God sends your way to be a blessing to you.

Trust God that when a situation doesn't work out with one person, that God has already put in place someone else as a ram in the bush to stand in the gap and take care of you.

That's something I had to learn through this whole ordeal myself. I'm so used to being a hands-on type person who's always in control that I have to remember to keep God in the driver's seat in my life.

If something doesn't work out a certain way as I had planned, I have to remember that all things work together for good for them that love God and that are called according to His purpose *(Romans 8:28)*. Often when things don't work out one way they work out a different way and I have to trust God through the process. And what process is that? The process of continuing to order my steps and lead me to that promised land that He has for me.

And He has one for you, too.

Whatever your ultimate destiny is in Him, whatever it is you desire, God wants to take you there, but He wants you to trust Him along the way.

No matter what obstacles, temptations or bumps, bruises or storms you may face along the way, God still wants to lead and guide you to that special place in Him.

God says in His Word:

Let not your heart be troubled: ye believe in God, believe also in me. John 14:1

The word, *troubled*, translated from the Greek means, agitated, anxious or restless, and the word, *believe*, means to place confidence and trust in Jesus.

So God doesn't want our heart to be anxious, agitated or restless, instead He wants us to place our total confidence and trust in the Lord, Jesus Christ.

When we trust Him, we freely give Him the driver's seat of our lives while knowing everything is going to be alright in Him.

And that's where I am now, six months later.

I can honestly say that this whole ordeal has made me more confident in the God I serve and the fact that He is for me.

I feel like with Him I can do anything, accomplish anything, and since the accident I feel like if I wanted to jump twenty feet, I can now jump forty. I now truly that believe that nothing, NOTHING is too hard for God and that with Him on my side we can do great things together for His kingdom to advance His message of Christ's love and make a difference in this world together.

Six months later, I can not only walk, I can jump, I can dance, I can shout and I can sing.

I have a new song in my heart and a new pep in my step.

And as a result of going through, I can truly say it's ONLY by the grace of God that I'm standing here today, and that with Him I can run on another hundred miles.

Just like the song says, the song I played on YouTube every day at least once during my two-week hospital stay . . . I been running for Jesus a long time and I'm not tired yet!

Trust in the LORD with all thine heart; and lean not unto thine own understanding. In all thy ways acknowledge him, and he shall direct thy paths. Be not wise in thine own eyes: fear the LORD, and depart from evil. It shall be health to thy navel, and marrow to thy bones. Proverbs 3:5-8

CHAPTER 26

FACING MY FEARS

Sunday, September 20

So the other week, during prayer the Lord led me to rejoin the praise team at a ministry I'm a part of and have been for a couple years – Global Empowerment Ministries. It's been six months since I was up on that stage ministering to others with the team and I will admit I grew comfortable setting it aside for now. But now that my leg is healing well, and that I can stand up longer without feeling the pain as much, then returning shouldn't be too bad.

Or so I thought.

On the way to rehearsal yesterday, as I looked forward to the return, suddenly on the way there tears welled in my eyes and I cried hysterically. Then it hit me. The real reason I hadn't returned to the praise team before now, was because of fear!

You see, the accident happened last March right after leaving the church after praise team rehearsal. I had thought I buried that fear and my upset from it, but driving to praise team rehearsal somehow reminded me of the pain I experienced that fateful day. And when I entered the church and saw everyone sincerely glad for my return, that made me cry even more.

So I viewed yesterday as the day I decided to face my fear, and now today, Sunday, I was able to praise and worship God with the team and usher in the presence of God while telling the Lord "Thank You" for all He's brought me from. It was a wonderful feeling to know I serve a God who, since He was the one who initiated my return, knew exactly why I needed to return in the first place. He knew I needed to face my fear, and He put it right in front of me. It was as if He was saying, "I'm not going to let you off this easy. I have called you for such a time as this to do this work in this season and use your gift in music to bless this house, and I'm not going to let any devil in hell rob you of my being able to use you to usher in my Glory."

So thank You, Daddy, for allowing me to face my fear and bind it in the name of Jesus. Praising You this morning reminded me of the real reason I was there in the first place – to glorify You and usher in Your presence for Your people and to set the table for the Word which is to come.

It's never been about me. It's about God using me, even in this, for His glory. And when He's glorified, I'm satisfied.

So what is it that you have to face and haven't done so yet because of fear? Has God called you to go back to that place of pain so you can regain your strength and your peace and your joy? Is there a previous relationship with a friend or loved one that may have ended on a sour note and God is calling you to go back and apologize to them? I know they may have been the most in the wrong, but if God is calling you to go back – He's doing it for a reason. He's doing it to free you from the painful grip of fear that may have a hold on you. He's doing it so you can be freed to move forward with His plan and perfect will for your life. Sometimes, in the middle of a storm, not only will we face giants along the way, we also have to bind fear, in Jesus' name and step up to the plate and tell the devil, "Take that," while ushering in a few more . . . a few more souls . . . a few more books . . . a few more sermons . . . a few more anointed business deals . . . a few more of whatever it is God has called you to do.

I remember when Jesus walked in temporary fear, as He was about to go to the cross to die for our sins. While He had every intention on doing the right thing, He knew that as God on the earth yet still a man on the earth who feels pain and will feel the sting of death for a moment as He takes on our sins on the cross, He knew it was going to feel bad. He knew it was going to hurt! So, out of fear, as his sweat was like drops of blood because of how nervous and afraid He was in the Garden of Gethsemane (Luke 22:44), He asked His Heavenly Father.

And he went a little farther, and fell on his face, and prayed, saying, *O my Father, if it be possible, let this cup pass from me . . . nevertheless not as I will, but as thou wilt. Matthew 26:39a*

He was so troubled that he fell on his face and prayed. He asked God for another way, another way to accomplish the same goal of saving the world from their sins – another method. He knew God was Sovereign and that the plan was already in place and that His purpose was already made known to Him, but Jesus, at that very moment, wanted a way out and an escape from the pain he was about to experience.

Jesus was full of pain; he struggled hard in prayer. Sweat dripped from his face like drops of blood falling to the ground. *Luke 22:44*

So it's not a sin to have a moment of weakness or feel pain. Even Jesus did. The key is to go to God with your pain and seek the Lord in prayer so He can turn pain and fear into renewed promise and fearless favor. Jesus knew what He had to do, and because God called Him He knew He was equipped to do it . . . He just needed that extra dose of faith which He received in prayer to remind Him of who He is and for which He came.

So while in prayer, His initial trepidation was turned around as He boldly declared, "nevertheless not as I will, but as thou wilt." *(Matthew 26:39b)*

That's when He realized it wasn't about Him. *That's* when He remembered who His master and His maker was. *That's* when He remembered who *He* was – sent, chosen and predestined by God to save the world.

So whatever you're going through, even while afraid, take the time to face the fear by going to God in prayer and allowing Him to remind you who of who you are.

Allow Him to remind you that you are more than a conqueror, that you are the head and not the tail, and that you can do all things through Christ who strengthens you. Remind yourself that when you are weak, there you are strong, because you go in His favor, in His power, in His anointing and in His Grace. You go in His Name.

So face your fears, even through the tears, and come out fighting like the champion you already are, remembering that the battle has already been fought and the victory has already been won.

Now thanks be unto God, which always causeth us to tri-umph in Christ, and maketh manifest the savour of his knowledge by us in every place. 2 Corinthians 2:14

And he said unto me, My grace is sufficient for thee: for my strength is made perfect in weakness. Most gladly therefore will I rather glory in my infirmities, that the power of Christ may rest upon me. 2 Corinthians 12:9

CHAPTER 27

NEW MOUNTAIN

Saturday, September 26
"*So go down and breathe through your nose. Take a deep breath first, or you can hum while in the water and that automatically causes you to breathe through your nose.*"

I'm excited because today was the first day of my new undertaking since the accident – I'm learning how to swim!

I've always wanted to learn, especially since I almost drowned twice. I remember on one occasion I was at a family water park in the wave pool and I floated over to eight feet of water while on an inflated tube, waving to my friends who were ashore several feet in front of me. Next thing you know the wave bell rang and crashed through, and my tube toppled over so I, recklessly, started waving my hands for someone to grab me so I wouldn't drown.

Eventually a young girl who looked to be about only eleven years old with long, blond hair came and got me and carried me over to the side. She was a brave soul. Soon after the rescue the lifeguard made an announcement, "If you cannot swim, do not go out to eight feet of water." Was he coming for me? (lol) I knew that was a suggestion to others who may think about doing something crazy as I did. Don't ask me why I did it. Not thinking, I guess. Funny thing is, I realized something about each time I almost drowned (first time I was about six years old and went to reach for a ball at the YMCA and slipped and fell in the water. A Girl Scout member scooped me up). I knew without a shadow of a doubt, that I would be saved. I have this weird relationship with the water, where I truly believe it to be my friend. In my twenties I even rode Jet Skis all the way across the lake to a separate island. When I told my dad what I did he almost fell over, because he knew I couldn't swim. "How could you do that?" he asked. He couldn't fathom taking a risk on something which may result in a loss of life. However I never looked at it like that. Drowning never came to my mind; I just knew I wanted to Jet Ski and that it sounded like fun.

So now, thanks to the grace of God, He's kept me both times, but now it's time to learn how to swim on my own so I can save someone else who may be drowning lol.

My doctor says swimming would be good for me; for my femur especially. I've also heard swimming works every muscle and that it's a great workout. And since I love water and being in it, I view it as therapeutic as well.

I said all this to say, no matter what challenge you may be going through right now, part of the battle is all in how you look at it.

As the saying goes, you can make a mountain out of a molehill. For example, in those instances where I almost drowned I could've gone berserk and starting kicking and screaming and fighting against anyone who tried to help me, but instead I just made my request for help known (by flailing my arms in the air every time my body went up from the waves) and simply waited for someone to come get me.

That's the beginner lesson, or, like the babe in Christ. Waiting for a pastor or someone to feed them the milk of the Word, or the good parts that taste good.

Eventually it's time to move on from milk to meat. Eventually it's time to move on from being helped, to working toward being able to help others. Eventually it's time to take all the pain you've been through in your storm and use that to help someone else and free someone else.

So I'm excited about my swim lessons. Another black eye for the devil. Not only am I walking again, I can now dance, I can now jump, I can now run, and now I'm learning how to swim. Take that, devil.

Submit yourselves therefore to God. Resist the devil, and he will flee from you. James 4:7

As newborn babes, desire the sincere milk of the word, that ye may grow thereby:
*   If so be ye have tasted that the Lord is gracious. 1 Peter 2:2-3*

CONCLUSION

This whole ordeal with the car accident has definitely been an eye-opener. I'm definitely thankful to God for allowing me to go through it, because it has blessed me in so many ways (Yes, I said the car accident blessed me). It has blessed me to know that I truly am more than a conqueror through Christ, as He has literally caused me to overcome. It has blessed me in that it made my relationship with God that much stronger and drew me closer to Him as I relied on Him, in a very real sense, for everything from seeing me through during the dark nights of the hospital stay, to helping me overcome any fears, to making sure all goes well with the procedure and the surgery to literally causing new bone to grow inside my body in order to heal it and to recover me, and bringing me to a point of healing and continued recovery as I continue to get stronger and stronger with every physical therapy session.

I now realize where my strength and my help comes from. Many say they know where their help comes from, but until they go through something, they're not always able to experience the realness of that statement. When I was sick in my body – my help came from the Lord. When the doctor said it could take one to two years for my leg to recover – my help came from the Lord. When the doctor said there was a possibility that my bone won't unionize and grow inside in order to heal – my help came from the Lord. And even when others said I would be bound to a life of limping and leaning over; I now walk tall, with my head held high; for my help came from the Lord.

I now know the true meaning of the Lord being my very best friend. I feel like, with Him on my side, I can literally do anything I set my hands to because He said He would prosper it. I can run through a troop and leap over walls because He said He would give me the strength to do it. I can bless and impact thousands, if not millions of lives with the gospel of Jesus Christ and the saving and delivering power of our Lord because He would do it through me.

I feel like the servant, Isaiah, who told God, "Here am I; send me." Whatever You want me to do; I'll do. Wherever You want me to go; I'll go. I'm not playing either, Jesus. Since you've given me a second chance at life; I want to make it count. I want to make my life count to countless others who, at the end of the day, will know that Jesus is Lord and that He cares about you.

So no matter what you're going through, know that it's not a struggle, it's a fight. But it's a fixed fight, because while you go through, and watch and pray as the Scripture says, know that God is already working behind the scenes and that you've already won. How would you act if you knew that whatever you were going through right now, that there was already victory on the other side? If you're facing health challenges, how would you act if He healed you today? If you're struggling financially, how you act if He came through with a financial breakthrough for you today? Suffering the loss of a loved one, how would you act if God, Himself, wrapped His loving arms around you and told you it was going to be all okay, today?

So no matter what you're going through, no matter what your "broken place" may be, know that God is with you, He's in you to strengthen you, and that you're not alone. He's all you need to achieve success, and all the success comes from you and there's nothing you can do to earn it . . . all you have to do is receive it.

I now understand the Scripture when it says:

My brethren, count it all joy when ye fall into divers temptations;
Knowing this, that the trying of your faith worketh patience.
But let patience have her perfect work, that ye may be perfect and entire, wanting nothing. James 1:2-4

So if you're seemingly facing obstacles and challenges on every side, count it all joy. Laugh in the devil's face – why, because God says when your faith is tried your patience is activated which leads to your perfection and maturity in Christ which causes you to open your eyes and realize that with God you have everything you need and you want for absolutely nothing.

To God be the Glory!

Who shall separate us from the love of Christ? Shall tribulation, or distress, or persecution, or famine, or nakedness, or peril, or sword? As it is written, For thy sake we are killed all the day long; we are accounted as sheep for the slaughter. Nay, in all these things we are more than conquerors through him that loved us. For I am persuaded, that neither death, nor life, nor angels, nor principalities, nor powers, nor things present, nor things to come. Nor height, nor depth, nor any other creature, shall be able to separate us from the love of God, which is in Christ Jesus our Lord.
Romans 8:35-39

I pray this book blessed you, if so, be a blessing by posting a review online and encouraging others to receive their own copy and be blessed and encouraged by it as well.

Continued blessings, and, as always, be and *STAY* encouraged!

SPECIAL INVITATIONS

If you have never accepted Jesus Christ as your personal Lord and Savior, I would like to invite you to receive Him in your heart today.

Romans 10:9-10 states:

That if thou shall confess with thy mouth the Lord Jesus, and shalt believe in thine heart that God hath raised him from the dead, thou shalt be saved. For with the heart man believeth unto righteousness; and with the mouth confession is made unto salvation.

Now recite this prayer out loud:

"Father, God, I believe that Jesus Christ is the Son of God. I believe He died for me, carried my sins for me, and that He arose, and is alive right now. Lord, Jesus, come into my heart. I repent of sin, and I turn toward You. I receive You as my Savior, and I confess

You as my Lord. I thank You, Lord, that according to Your Word, I am born again. In Jesus' Name, Amen."

Praise God, you are now saved! Though you still look the same on the outside, on the inside you are a new creature in Christ according to *2 Corinthians 5:17*.

If you do not have a church home, I encourage you to join and become active in one that teaches the Word of God so that you will continue to grow spiritually.

When it comes to choosing a church home, go where you grow!

Remember this day forever as your "born-again Birthday" as today marks a day of new beginnings for you!

\-\-

If you're already saved, I would like to extend another invitation to you. If, since you've been saved, you've fallen away from God or been out of fellowship with Him where you know you need to repent from some things in your past, I'd like you to recite this prayer:

"Father God, please forgive me for I have sinned. Your Word says that if I confess my sins then you are faithful and just to forgive me of my sins and cleans me of all unrighteousness. Please forgive me for (state the sins), and also any place in my heart where I have missed the mark. Thank You for honoring Your Word and bringing me back in right standing with You as I have confessed my sin, with the heart intention of not doing it again.

"Thank You for the shed blood of Jesus which has washed away my sin and has brought me back in right standing with You as I continue and strive to be the godly person You have called and predestined me to be. In Jesus' Name, Amen."

Praise God, you are cleansed of all past sins! You are whole! You are back in right standing with God.

You are now free to worship and praise God freely, lifting up holy hands without wrath or doubting according to *1 Timothy 2:8*. Remember, if you ever miss the mark, always run *to* God, never *away* from God, and He'll be standing right there with open arms, ready to receive you once again.

ABOUT THE AUTHOR

Award-winning author, licensed minister, national speaker and songwriter Kim Brooks is the founder of Kim Brooks Ministries International and Driven Enterprises, LLC headquartered in her hometown of Detroit, MI.

A Michigan State grad, Kim is the national bestselling author of novels, *She That Findeth, He's Fine...But is He Saved?* and its sequel, *He's Saved...But is He For Real?* and self-help books *How To Date and Stay Saved, The Little Black Survival Book for Single Saints* and more.

An abstinence until marriage advocate, which is not only her speaking platform but also her testimony, Kim has been a guest columnist for *Gospel Today* and featured on numerous media including Totally Christian Television and The Word Network. She also publishes a monthly eNewsletter, *The Single Heart,* and an online daily devotional that encourages thousands globally and is subscribable for free on her blog, Kimontheweb.com

ADDITIONAL TITLES BY KIM BROOKS

<u>Non-fiction</u>

How To Date and Stay Saved

The Little Black Survival Book for Single Saints

Is It a Sin To Masturbate: What the Bible Says Revealed, Know and Be Free

The Ultimate Guide to Christian Online Dating

Get Over Your Ex in One Weekend

Kim Brooks

Fiction

She That Findeth

He's Fine...But is He Saved?

He's Saved...But is He For Real?

FOLLOW KIM ONLINE

Facebook: http://www.facebook.com/kimbrooksofficialpage

Twitter: http://www.Twitter.com/kimontheweb

Instagram: http://www.Instagram.com/kimontheweb

"How To Date and Stay Saved" Monthly Podcast: http://www.blogtalkradio.com/kimbrooks (also on iTunes)

Blog: http://www.kimontheweb.com/blog

Subscribe to Kim's YouTube Channel at http://www.YouTube.com/kimontheweb

Subscribe to Kim's free eNewsletter and daily devotional at http://www.KimOnTheWeb.com